Diet drink

Protecting Your Everyday Wellness with Peace of Mind

By

SHARON BARTON

Table of Contents

Chapter 1

Chapter 2

Chapter 3

Chapter 4

Chapter 5

Chapter 6

Chapter 7

Introduction

In a world where our health and well-being are paramount, we are confronted with countless options to improve our daily routines. From the food we eat to the beverages we choose, it is critical to prioritize safety and peace of mind.

Unfortunately, not all diet drinks on the market offer the same level of assurance. Some obscure brands may unknowingly pose risks to our health, raising concerns about their potential dangers.

Chapter 1

Diet Drinks Explained

Diet drinks are beverages that are specifically formulated to be low in or completely devoid of calories, sugar, or carbohydrates; they are frequently marketed as low-calorie or zero-calorie alternatives to regular sugary beverages, aiming to provide a lower-calorie or zero-calorie option for individuals looking to reduce their sugar intake, manage their weight, or control their blood sugar levels.

The term "diet drinks" is sometimes used as an umbrella word to describe a range of beverage types with zero or decreased calories, such as diet sodas, diet teas, diet energy drinks, and flavored water, the particular composition and components of which vary depending on the brand and product.

There are several sorts of diet drinks on the market, each with its own set of qualities and compositions.

Diet Beverages

Diet sodas are carbonated beverages that taste similar to ordinary sodas but include artificial sweeteners instead of sugar. They are available in a variety of flavors, including cola, lemon-lime, orange, and others.

Energy Drinks on a Diet

Diet energy drinks, like regular energy drinks, provide a burst of energy but with fewer or no calories, and they often contain artificial sweeteners, caffeine, and additional components such as B vitamins and herbal extracts.

Iced Teas on a Diet

Diet iced teas are manufactured by substituting artificial sweeteners for sugar to provide a sweet taste without the added calories, and they come in a variety of flavors such as lemon, peach, raspberry, and green tea.

Water with Flavor

Flavored water products are frequently promoted as diet drinks since they have few to no calories or sugar, and they are typically infused with natural or artificial tastes, with some also including electrolytes or vitamins.

Water with a Sparkle

Sparkling water, also known as carbonated water or soda water, is available in diet versions that use artificial sweeteners or natural flavors to provide a refreshing and fizzy drink without added sugars or calories; it is available in a variety of flavors and is occasionally combined with fruit essences or extracts.

Fruit Juices on a Diet

These are fruit juices that have had their sugar content lowered or abolished by employing artificial sweeteners or natural sugar alternatives, with the goal of providing the flavor of typical fruit juices without the high sugar content.

Chapter 2

The Truth About Diet Soda

It causes additional weight gain.

Many people who wished to lose weight would substitute diet soda for ordinary soda, only to be surprised when they not only failed to lose weight, but actually gained more!

So, what role does diet soda play in weight gain?

While diet soda does not contain real sugar or calories, it does contain a lot of additives and artificial ingredients, including sweeteners, which are full of unnatural chemicals that can cause your body to crave more high-calorie and sugar-laden foods. Artificial sweeteners may also confuse your body into miscalculating the number of calories you are actually consuming, causing your metabolism to slow down and making it more difficult to lose weight.

It has been associated with type 2 diabetes.

Diet soda's artificial sweeteners can actually produce a spike in blood sugar and insulin levels, which can lead to diabetic shock in people who already have diabetes.

Diet soda can induce weight gain and a decreased metabolic rate, which can be the start of a formula for diabetes in the future.

It has the potential to induce heart problems.

Diet soda has been linked to an increased risk of heart problems such as congestive heart failure, heart disease, and/or heart attacks.
It contains artificial sweeteners, including aspartame, and other health concerns associated with diet soda

intake, such as weight gain, higher blood sugar levels, and diabetes, can all contribute to cardiac problems.

It can virtually double your chances of suffering a stroke.

This risk is primarily caused by a high sodium intake, which can cause an increase in heart rate and blood pressure, which can lead to blood clots in the brain. The amount of sodium in a can of diet soda varies depending on the flavor and brand. On the low side, you can expect to drink 12 milligrams of sodium, while on the high side, that number can be more than 5 times as high.

Weight control

Diet soda can be a beneficial tool for weight management since it is a low-calorie alternative to regular soda, which is heavy in sugar. By drinking diet soda instead of regular soda, people can reduce their overall calorie consumption, potentially assisting with weight loss or weight maintenance efforts.

Appetite and Cravings

Artificial sweeteners may increase cravings for sweet foods or disrupt appetite regulation, potentially undermining weight management efforts.

Dental Care

Diet soda, like regular soda, is acidic and, when drank frequently or in excessive quantities, can lead to dental erosion and tooth decay. To maintain dental health, it is best to limit soda consumption generally and practice good oral hygiene routines.

IndividualVariations

People's reactions to diet soda can vary depending on factors such as heredity, overall diet quality, lifestyle behaviors, and personal preferences. Some people may find diet soda beneficial in their weight loss efforts, while others may prefer to avoid it owing to concerns or personal preferences.

Chapter 3

Why Is Diet Soda Worse Than Regular Soda?

Aside from weight gain, persons who consume diet soda are more likely to acquire heart disease; drinking just one diet soda per day increases your risk of acquiring high blood sugar, blood pressure, and cholesterol by 36%.

Soda is a major contributor to the present "obesity epidemic," and it has even been connected to an increased risk of asthma.

One of the main reasons why some of us still drink regular coke is that it tastes fantastic without the weird aftertaste seen in diet sodas, and it is also the favored soda choice for folks who do not want to consume the artificial sugar substitutes found in diet sodas.

It is impossible to say definitively that one is better than the other because each has its own set of advantages and disadvantages;

nonetheless, regardless of which one you choose, keep in mind that neither is beneficial for your health.

Chapter 4

What Effect Do Diet Drinks Have on Weight Loss?

Diet beverages should not be viewed as a quick fix for weight loss.

Diet beverages, also known as low-calorie or zero-calorie drinks, are frequently taken as part of a weight loss or calorie-restricted diet;

nevertheless, the actual impact of diet drinks on weight control is a source of disagreement among specialists.

Calorie Cutting

Diet drinks are often sweetened with artificial sweeteners, which provide a sweet taste without adding significant calories; by replacing diet drinks for ordinary sugary beverages, you can reduce your overall calorie intake, which may aid to weight loss.

Cravings and Appetite

Consuming diet beverages may enhance sensations of hunger or cravings for sweet foods, as artificial sweeteners can be considerably sweeter than sugar, thereby offsetting the calorie reduction achieved by choosing diet drinks.

Psychological Aspects

ingesting a diet drink may produce the perception of "saving calories," which might impact eating patterns; nevertheless, some people may compensate for the calorie reduction from diet beverages by ingesting more calories from other sources, which can sabotage weight loss efforts.

Effects on Metabolic Rate

The effect of artificial sweeteners on metabolism is currently unknown. Artificial sweeteners may interfere with the body's capacity to control calorie intake, perhaps leading to weight gain or metabolic dysregulation over time.

Individual Differences

Individual responses to diet drinks can vary greatly; some people may experience weight loss or improved weight management when including diet drinks in their diet, while others may not see any significant changes. Individual responses are influenced by factors such as genetics, overall diet, physical activity, and personal preferences.

Chapter 5

Blood Sugar and Diet Soda

In the near run, artificial sweeteners will not raise your blood sugar levels.

A can of diet coke, for example, will not trigger a blood sugar spike.

Diet soda has been linked to weight gain and metabolic syndrome, which can worsen or raise the risk of developing diabetes.

Diet soda is typically sweetened with artificial sweeteners such as aspartame or sucralose, which do not contain or have a minimal impact on blood sugar levels, making it suitable for people who are trying to manage their blood sugar levels or following a low-carbohydrate diet.

It's important to note, however, that there are several factors that can affect blood sugar levels, including overall diet, individual metabolism, and insulin response. Some studies suggest that consuming artificial sweeteners may still have an indirect effect on blood sugar control by potentially influencing appetite, cravings, and overall food choices.

If you have specific concerns about diet soda and your blood sugar levels, you should always speak with a healthcare practitioner or a certified dietitian who can provide specialized advice based on your specific health situation.

Chapter 6

Diet drink consumption psychological considerations

Diet drink psychological aspects can have a substantial impact on people's tastes, behaviors, and general connection with these beverages.

Health Advantages

Many people prefer diet beverages to ordinary sugary drinks because they believe they are a healthier alternative. The belief that diet drinks can help with weight loss or contribute to a more balanced diet might affect people's choices and consumption patterns.

Preferences in Taste

Personal taste preferences can heavily influence the decision to consume diet drinks. Some people may genuinely enjoy the taste of diet drinks, while others may develop a preference for them due to their lower sugar content or different flavor profiles.

Psychological Satisfaction and Reward

Diet beverages can provide a sense of fulfillment and satisfaction, especially for people aiming to limit their calorie or sugar intake; the feeling of indulging in a sweet-tasting beverage without the associated guilt or weight impact can contribute to pleasant psychological experiences.

Addiction or psychological dependence

Due to their taste, caffeine content, or habitual consumption patterns, some people may develop a psychological dependence on diet drinks. As with other beverages, the routines, associations, and emotional aspects surrounding diet drink consumption can create psychological ties that make it difficult to reduce or eliminate their intake.

Psychological Preparation

Positive messaging about health, fitness, and weight management may persuade individuals to pick diet drinks, associating them with healthier lifestyles and personal goals, according to advertising, marketing, and societal messages.

Factors of Emotion

In response to stress, boredom, or emotional pain, people may turn to diet beverages as a coping technique or emotional crutch; the act of sipping a diet drink can provide comfort or distraction, leading to emotional associations and addictions.

Peer Influence and Social Norms

Peer influence, cultural norms, or the desire to fit in with a specific group may influence individuals' choices and consumption patterns, and the perceived social acceptability or desirability of diet drinks can shape their consumption behaviors.

Individual experiences and psychological aspects might vary greatly; some people may have favorable experiences and health results with diet drinks, while others may have different preferences or sensitivities that alter their interaction with these beverages.

Chapter 7

Selecting the Best Beverages

Choosing the correct beverages is critical for sticking to a balanced diet and reaching your weight-loss objectives.

Examine the Label

When selecting beverages, make it a practice to carefully study the labels, looking for information on serving size, calorie content, added sugars, artificial sweeteners, and other additives. Choose options with minimal or no added sugars and avoid those with too many calories or dangerous substances.

Water

Water should be your go-to hydration beverage because it has no calories, quenches thirst, and supports various bodily functions. Carry a reusable water bottle with you throughout the day to stay hydrated. If plain water bores you, infuse it with slices of fruits, herbs, or cucumber for a refreshing twist.

Diet and low-calorie beverages

If you prefer flavored beverages, choose low-calorie or diet versions, which are typically formulated to have fewer calories or sugar than their regular counterparts. However, be wary of artificial sweeteners and other additives. Moderation is key, and these drinks should be included as part of a balanced diet rather than being relied on excessively.

Coffee and tea without sugar

As long as you avoid adding too much sugar or cream, unsweetened tea and coffee can be healthy beverage options. Green tea, black tea, herbal teas, and black coffee (without additional sugar) are low-calorie options that can deliver antioxidants and a slight energy boost.

Juices that have been freshly squeezed

While fruit juices can be an excellent source of vitamins and minerals, they can also be heavy in calories and sugar. Choose freshly squeezed juices or ones with no added sugars. However, whole fruits are generally a better alternative because they provide fiber and are more satisfying.

Milk and Dairy Substitutes

Milk and dairy alternatives, such as almond milk or soy milk, can be healthful. Choose low-fat or skim milk to limit calorie intake while still getting vital minerals like calcium and vitamin D. Flavored dairy alternatives should be avoided because they may contain additional sugars.

Limit your intake of sugary drinks.

Sugary beverages, such as soda, sports drinks, energy drinks, and sweetened fruit drinks, should be consumed in moderation or avoided entirely because they are high in calories, added sugars, and provide little nutritional value. Instead, choose water, herbal tea, or sparkling water with a splash of natural fruit juice.

Water is always the best choice for hydration; however, if you like other beverages, choose ones that are low in calories, added sugars, and artificial chemicals. Balance is important, and including a range of healthy beverages into your diet can contribute to overall wellness.

Conclusion

The desire to enhance one's well-being and health can take many different forms, including the desire for better health, increased awareness of good options, and protection from dangerous components.

Your diet will not benefit nutritionally from diet soda, and not all selections are reduced in calories or sugar. It's crucial to eat them in moderation and to be aware of any potential health risks linked to artificial sweeteners because they may also contribute to certain health conditions. emphasizing a healthy, diversified diet and frequent exercise.

www.ingramcontent.com/pod-product-compliance
Lightning Source LLC
Chambersburg PA
CBHW060857260726
48661CB00008B/3314